Part

Time

Diet

By Maria Phelps

The author and publisher are in no way responsible for misuse of this material.

Contact Information:

Maria Phelps

Mariaphelps5@yahoo.com

Author Photo was taken by Alexxus from AlexxusImaging.com

Foreword:

This will be the only diet you will ever need. You will not believe how quickly the weight will come off and stay off. You will be amazed at how much better you will feel physically and mentally. All of this without crazy diet scams, drinks, pills or exercise.

My Story:

When I got pregnant with my first child back in 1989, I gained almost 80lbs. Needless to say that when I had her, I only lost 25lbs. Then got pregnant with my 2nd child and gained 55lbs. I had lost weight after I had my 2nd child but still had a lot of extra weight on. According to those charts at the doctors' office, I was always at least 40lbs over weight. Not that I have a lot of faith in those charts but it always had a way of making me feel horrible about myself. Then, when I was 35, I had another child. Everyone knows the older you get, the harder it is to lose weight. Well, I had quite a bit to lose.

Every day I would wake up and constantly criticize the way I looked. I hated to look in the mirror. I would beat myself up emotionally about the way I looked. I never looked in the mirror and was happy with what I saw. When I would see myself in pictures (which was even worse) I had to accept that, that was the real me. I avoided anyone taking pictures of me. I just couldn't stand to look at myself in pictures. But, one day, my mother-in-law wanted to get a picture of my husband and I and our little girl, Lilyahna. She then brought us a copy of this picture and I kept it. I kept looking at that picture and thinking, "My God, Look at me!". It just drove me nuts to see myself in that picture.

One day, I woke up and looked in the mirror and literally said out loud, "That's it!!! I can't stand looking like this anymore. God, you have got to help me! Please help me lose weight!"

The next day I woke up with a great plan. And, that is the plan I am going to share with you.

First, I would like to share the picture that my mother-in-law had taken of me.

This was me in February of 2008. I am not sure what I weighed in this picture. I did not start my diet for another 2 months after this picture had been taken.

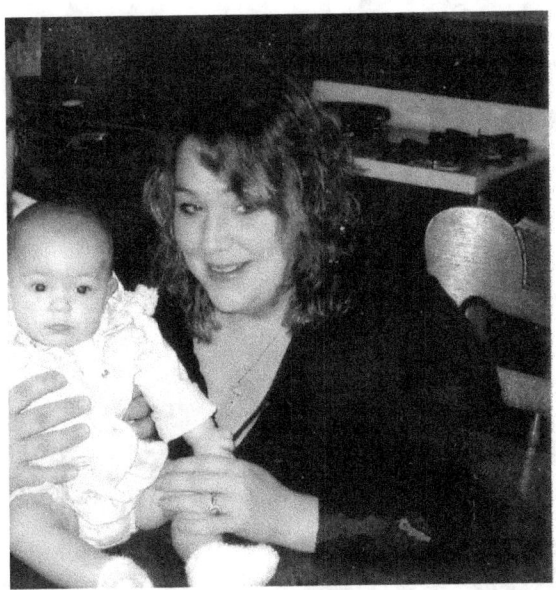

December 2008

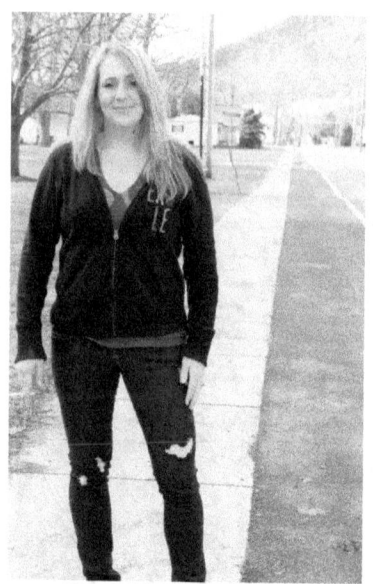

I lost 58lbs in 14 weeks on this diet. After a year and half off of this diet, I only gained 1 lb back. I also want to add that I own a Pizzeria. I had the temptations every day for all of the yummy food that I make there.

If I can do this… **Anyone** can do it!! I just keep telling myself that I wanted to be skinny. I wanted to be healthier. When I started this diet, my cholesterol was 290. After I lost the weight, my cholesterol went down to 204. I did not take any medication to lower that. It was strictly from losing weight.

After I had lost the weight, I went back to eating all the food that I had eaten before I went on the diet. I was eating pizza, wings and breadsticks and all that stuff that I used to eat before I went on my diet.

So, I want to share with you exactly how
I did it. I know that you will have just
as must success as I did.

The Diet:

There are a few things things that you are going to need for this diet

1. Tablet
2. Pencil or Pen
3. Lots of Willpower

First, let's take a look at what the "Healthcare Professionals" say you should weigh.

The following are a standard chart but they do vary from doctor to doctor. This is only a guideline to go by. Every person is shaped differently and your goal weight should be based on what makes you feel good about yourself and is a healthy weight.

STANDARD WEIGHT CHART FOR MEN

Height In Feet & Inches	Small Frame	Medium Frame	Large Frame
5'2"	128-134	131-141	138-150
5'3"	130-136	133-143	140-153
5'4"	132-138	135-145	142-156
5'5"	134-140	137-148	144-160
5'6"	136-142	139-151	146-164
5'7"	138-145	142-154	149-168
5'8"	140-148	145-157	152-172
5'9"	142-151	148-160	155-176
5'10"	144-154	151-163	158-180
5'11"	146-157	154-166	161-184
6'0"	149-160	157-170	164-188
6'1"	152-164	160-174	168-192
6'2"	155-168	164-178	172-197
6'3"	158-172	167-182	176-202
6'4"	162-176	171-187	181-207

STANDARD WEIGHT CHART FOR WOMEN

Height In Feet & Inches	Small Frame	Medium Frame	Large Frame
4'10"	102-111	109-121	118-131
4'11"	103-113	111-123	120-134
5'0"	104-115	113-126	122-137
5'1"	106-118	115-129	125-140
5'2"	108-121	118-132	128-143
5'3"	111-124	121-135	131-147
5'4"	114-127	124-138	134-151
5'5"	117-130	127-141	137-155
5'6"	120-133	130-144	140-159
5'7"	123-136	133-147	143-163
5'8"	126-139	136-150	146-167
5'9"	129-142	139-153	149-170
5'10"	132-145	142-156	152-173
5'11"	135-148	145-159	155-176
6'0"	138-151	148-162	158-179

The secret to this diet is: You don't diet every day. You diet for 2 days and then on the third day, you eat whatever you want. YES…whatever you want. If you want 3 candy bars and a bowl of ice cream…you can have it. But only on your days off. But you have to go off the diet on the 3rd day. Then go back on for 2 days and go off for another day and just repeat this cycle.

I talked to my physician about this and the only thing that we could come up with was it tricks your metabolism. On traditional diets you lose weight for the first 2 days and then it will taper off. On this diet, just when your body thinks it isn't going to get any more "fattening" food, it goes into starvation mode. Your metabolism starts to slow down. Then on the third day when you eat all the foods that you would normally eat, your body is fooled into thinking that you aren't on a diet anymore. Then when you go back on the diet the next day, you will keep losing the weight.

It is all about the calorie intake. Our body burns a certain amount of calories per day depending on what type of activity we are doing. Your body even burns calories when you're sleeping. So, the obvious thing to do is take in less calories than you can burn off in a day.

Here is a calorie burning chart

ACTIVITY	CALORIES USED:
Sleeping	60 per hour
Sitting on Couch	75 per hour
Grocery Shopping	90 per hour
Doing Light Household Chores	95 per hour
Standing in Line	100 per hour
Playing with Your Dog	115 per hour
Playing with Kids (not rigorous)	120 per hour
Driving	120 per hour
Shopping	135 per hour
Eating	140 per hour
Bowling	145 per hour
Household Chores (vacuuming or scrubbing)	225 per hour
Yoga (breaking a sweat)	230 per hour

Walking	230 per hour
Gardening	230 per hour
Brisk Walking	250 per hour
Playing Golf (riding in a golf cart)	250 per hour
Softball	260 per hour
Dancing	270 per hour
Skateboarding	275 per hour
Mowing the lawn (push mower)	295 per hour
Lifting Weights	300 per hour
Playing Golf (walking w/ bag)	330 per hour
Volleyball	340 per hour
Hiking	390 per hour
Shoveling Snow	400 per hour
Power Walking	400 per hour
Playing Basketball or Racquetball	510 per hour
Tennis	510 per hour

Swimming	520 per hour
Bicycling (fast pace)	530 per hour
Circuit Weight Training	540 per hour
Hiking	540 per hour
Stairclimber in a Gym	600 per hour
Jogging (5 miles per hour)	600 per hour
Running	700 per hour
Bicycling	710 per hour
Water Aerobics	720 per hour
Step Aerobics	750 per hour
Spinning Class in a Gym	820 per hour
Elliptical Rider or Rowing Machine	850 per hour
Jump Rope	900 per hour
Running (fast pace)	1000 per

The calorie intake for this diet is different for men and woman.

For men: You need to eat between 1700-1900 calories per day.

For women: You need to eat between 1200-1400 calories per day.

It really is that simple!

My philosophy:

The reason this diet works so good is, not only are you tricking your body but also your mind. When you are on a regular diet, you keep telling yourself, "I can't eat that, I am on a diet!" So, what I always told myself was, "I am going to have that on my day off!". Then I did. When we tell ourselves that we can't have something, we want it even more.

Another thing I did every night was envision the way I wanted to look. It kept me focused on my goal. I highly recommend doing this. It keeps your eye focused on the prize. Even though this diet is simple, it can be very hard to stick to when this world is full of wonderful fattening food everywhere you look.

In the following pages, I am going to give you some helpful little hints.

Helpful Hints:

1. Never eat something if you don't know how many calories are in it

2. Most of the fast food chains now have menus that have the calories of all their items.

3. Get a sufficient amount of sleep at night. When you are tired you have a tendency to eat sugary foods for energy.

4. Take a multivitamin.

5. Don't ever tell yourself you can't have something. Tell yourself...you don't want that right now.

6. Make sure when you are checking the calories in an item

that you also look at the serving size.

7. There are many sites on the web that provide a lot of low calorie meal options.

8. Have a dieting partner. You can get alot of emotional support from someone going through the same thing.

9. Please consult a physician before starting this diet to ensure you have no underlying health problems.

10. Set a goal date and stick to it.

11. The closer you get to your desired weight, your weight loss will slow down.

12. Keep telling yourself...I am eating to live NOT living to eat!

Sample menu

Breakfast: 4 slices of Lit'er bread with sugar free jelly   90 Calories

Snack: 1 cup of sugar free jello

                            20 calories

1 cup of grapes   62 calories

Lunch: Ham & Cheese sandwich with mustard.   195 calories

Banana   100 calories

Snack: 100 calorie pack popcorn with spray butter   100 calories

Dinner: "Hormel Compleats" 90 second meal   290 calories

Small can of vegetables   50 calories

Snack: Sugar Free pudding (made with skim milk) with fat free coolwhip and bananas   290 calories

This is 1200 calories. As you can see, I wasn't starving myself. It was all about the choices I made.

What I did was, go to the supermarket and read all the labels on my stuff and choose lower calorie items instead of the higher calorie items.

Encouraging Words

You can do this. It is hard for the first week but it gets easier. The more weight you lose, the easier it gets. The pounds were literally melting off of me and they will on you too as well. Think positive and keep your goal in mind. It does take willpower and dedication. But once you lose that first 5 pounds and still can eat all the foods you love 2-3 days a week. You will be hooked. I have included a calorie chart to make it even easier for you to follow this diet. I am also including a list of some of the items that I found were very helpful in my dieting process.

List of great diet foods:

1. Spray butter
2. Canned soup
3. Sugar-Free jello
4. Lit'er bread (walmart)
5. Sugar-Free pudding
6. Yogurt
7. Hormel "Compleats" meals
8. Lean Cuisines
9. Parmesan cheese
10. Spaghetti Sauce
11. Cooked Ham
12. Chicken (not fried)
13. Canned Potatoes
14. Vegetables
15. Fruits
16. 100 calorie packs
17. Ketchup & Mustard
18. Pam cooking spray

19. Low calorie cheese
20. Popcorn

This is just a small list but there are so many out there to choose from.

Websites with low calorie meal ideas

Foodnetwork.com

Delish.com

DinnerMadeEasy.com

Food.com

Eatingwell.com

Allrecipes.com

Cookinglight.com

Bettycrocker.com

These are just a few websites. There are so many more

Starting Weight_____

Goal Weight_____

Goal Date_____

	Pounds lost	Pounds to go
Week 1		
Week 2		
Week 3		
Week 4		
Week 5		
Week 6		
Week 7		
Week 8		

Week 9		
Week 10		
Week 11		
Week 12		
Week 13		
Week 14		
Week 15		
Week 16		

Good Luck!!!

Calorie chart

Alcohol	Serving Size	Calories
Beer, regular	12-ounce can or bottle	144
Beer, non-alcoholic	12-ounce can or bottle	60 to 90 (depending on brand)
Distilled gin, rum, vodka, & whiskey (80 proof)	1 ounce	65
Liqueur, coffee (53 proof)	1 ounce	117
Liqueur, creme de menthe (72 proof)	1 ounce	125
Wine, red	1 wine glass (4 ounces)	91
Wine, white	1 wine glass (4 ounces)	86
Wine, rose	1 wine glass (4 ounces)	90
Wine, dessert	3 ounces	130

Meats	Serving Size	Calories
Frankfurter, Beef	1 each	184
Ground Beef, extra lean (raw)	1 ounce	66
Ground Beef, extra lean (raw)	16 ounces (1 pound)	1056
Ground Beef, lean (raw)	1 ounce	75
Ground Beef, lean (raw)	16 ounces (1 pound)	1200
Ground Beef, regular (raw)	1 ounce	88
Ground Beef, regular (raw)	16 ounces (1 pound)	1408
Ground Beef, extra lean (broiled or grilled))	4 ounces (1/4 pound)	264
Ground Beef, lean (broiled or grilled)	4 ounces (1/4 pound)	290
Ground Beef, regular (broiled or grilled)	4 ounces (1/4 pound)	328
Pepperoni	1 ounce	148
	1 slice	27
Flank Steak (broiled or grilled)	1 ounce	43

	Serving Size	Calories
Porterhouse Steak, prime grade (broiled or grilled)	1 ounce 8 ounces	55 440
Sirloin Steak, lean (broiled or grilled)	1 ounce 8 ounces	53 427
Tenderloin Steak or Roast (broiled or grilled)	1 ounce 8 ounces	51 406
T-Bone Steak (broiled or grilled)	1 ounce 8 ounces	50 402

Breads	Serving Size	Calories
Bagel, plain	1 bagel	320
Bagel, cinnamon raisin	1 bagel	350
Bagel, egg	1 bagel	330
Bagel, onion	1 bagel	330
Bagel, poppyseed	1 bagel	360
Bagel, sesame	1 bagel	350
Bagel, whole wheat	1 bagel	360
Breads, all types, regular sliced	1 slice (1 ounce)	60 to 80
Bread, French and Sourdough	1 slice (1 ounce)	88

Bread Crumbs, plain (dry)	1 cup	120
Eggroll Wrapper	1 each	23
English Muffin, plain (inc. sourdough)	1 each	135
Panko breading	1/2 cup	110
Pita Bread, white, whole wheat	1 (6.5" diameter)	150
Spring Roll Skins or Wrappers (Rice Paper)	2 ounces	200
Won Ton Wrapper	1 each	23

Cereal	Serving Size	Calories
All Bran	1/2 cup	79.2
Cheerios	1 cup	109.5
Corn Flakes	1 cup	100
Corn Grits, white	1/4 cup uncooked	140

	1 cup cooked	145
Frosted Flakes	3/4 cup	119.2
Grape Nuts	1/2 cup	208
Kashi, puffed	3/4 cup	90
Rice Krispies	1 1/4 cups	124.4
Rolled Oats (Oatmeal), quick	1 cup cooked 1 cup uncooked	145 311
Raisin Bran	1 cup	186
Shredded Wheat	2 biscuits	156.4

Cheese	Serving Size	Calories
America, processed	1 ounce	106
Blue Cheese, Danish	1 ounce	100
Brie	1 ounce	85
Camembert	1 ounce	122

Cheddar, regular	1 ounce	114
Cheddar, low fat	1 ounce	80
Chevre	1 ounce	88
Cottage Cheese, regular	1/2 cup	117
Cottage Cheese, 2% low-fat	1/2 cup	100
Cottage Cheese, fat-free	1/2 cup	70
Cream Cheese, regular	1 ounce 3-ounce package	99 297
Cream Cheese, light or low fat	1 ounce	65
Cream Cheese, fat-free	1 ounce	27
Edam Cheese	1 ounce	101
Feta Cheese, cow or sheep	1 ounce	75
Fontina Cheese	1 ounce	110
Goat Cheese	1 ounce	103

Gorgonzota	1 ounce	109
Gouda	1 ounce	101
Gruyere	1 ounce	117.1
Havarti	1 ounce	117
Laughing Cow, Creamy Swiss, Light	1 wedge	35
Monterey Jack	1 ounce	106
Mozzarella, whole milk	1 ounce	80
Mozzarella, part skim, low moisture	1 ounce	79.4
Parmesan Cheese	1 ounce	111
Parmesan Cheese, grated	1 tablespoon	23
	1 ounce	129
Provolone	1 ounce	100
Ricotta, whole milk	1 ounce	49

Roquefort	1 ounce	102
Swiss	1 ounce	100
Tofu, raw	1 ounce	22
	1/2 cup	94
Tofu, firm	1 ounce	41
	1/2 cup	183

Chocolate	Serving Size	Calories
Chocolate, 62%, semi-sweet	1 ounce	140
Chocolate, dark, 70%,	1 ounce	170
bittersweet	1 ounce	180
Chocolate, extra dark, 82%	1 ounce	162
Chocolate, white	1 ounce	135
Chocolate, unsweetened (baking)	1 tablespoon	80
Chocolate Syrup,	2 tablespoons	133
Chocolate Syrup, light	2 tablespoons	50
Hot Fudge Topping, regular	2 tablespoons	100

Cocoa, dry powder, unsweetened	1 tablespoon	12
	1 cup	197

Coffee	Serving Size	Calories
Starbucks, Carmel Frappuccino Coffee, no whip	16 fluid ounces	280
Starbucks, Carmel Frappuccino Coffee, whip	16 fluid ounces	430
Starbucks, Carmel Frappuccino Coffee only	16 fluid ounces	260
Starbucks, Caffe Latte, non-fat milk	16 fluid ounces	165
Starbucks, Caffe Latte, whole milk	16 fluid ounces	260
Starbucks, Caffe au Lait, whole milk	16 fluid ounces	140

Starbucks, Caffe au Lait, non-fat milk	16 fluid ounces	90
Starbucks, Caffe Americano, whole milk	16 fluid ounces	15
Starbucks, Caffe Mocha, whole milk, whip	16 fluid ounces	400
Starbucks, Caffe Mocha, non-fat milk, whip	16 fluid ounces	330
Starbucks, Caffe Mocha, non-fat milk, no whip	16 fluid ounces	220
Starbucks, Cappuccino, whole milk	16 fluid ounces	150
Starbucks, Cappuccino, non-fat milk	16 fluid ounces	100

Baking	Serving Size	Calories
Baking Powder	1 teaspoon	8
Baking Soda	1 teaspoon	0
Beef Broth or Stock, fat-free	1 cup	16.8

Cornstarch	1 tablespoon	30
Cream of Mushroom Soup, 98% fat-free	1/2 cup	70
Cream of Mushroom Soup, regular	1/2 cup	100
Cream of Tartar	1 teaspoon	2
Gelatin, unflavored	1 package (Knox)	25
Gelatin, flavored, sugar-free	1 (.6-ounce) pkg	6
Horseradish. prepared	1 teaspoon	5
Ketchup (Catsup)	1 tablespoon	15
	1 cup	240
Mayonnaise, regular	1 tablespoon	100
Mayonnaise, light	1 tablespoon	50
Mayonnaise, reduced fat	1 tablespoon	20
Mayonnaise, fat free	1 tablespoon	11
Mayonnaise, Weight Watchers, light	1 tablespoon	50
Mustard, Dijon	1 tablespoon	18
Mustard, yellow	1 tablespoon	10

Olives, Kalamata, pitted	4 olives	45
Olives, Spanish, green with pimiento	2 olives	15
Onion Powder	1 teaspoon	5
Onion Salt	1 teaspoon	1
Onion Soup Mix, dry	1 package (4 tablespoons)	118
Nori, toasted seaweed	1 sheet	10
Pickle, bread & butter, slices	1 ounce	20
Pickle, dill	1 medium (3 3/4")	12
Pickle, sweet	1 large (3")	41
Pickle, relish sweet	1 tablespoon	21
Salsa	2 tablespoons	6
	1 cup	48
Sour Cream, regular	2 tablespoons (1 ounce)	61
Sour Cream, light	2 tablespoons (1 ounce)	40
Sour Cream, fat-free	2 tablespoons (1 ounce)	20
Soy Sauce	1 tablespoon	11
	1/4 cup	35

Vanilla Extract	1 teaspoon	10
Vinegar, cider	1 tablespoon	2
Vinegar, balsamic	1 tablespoon	5
Vinegar, raspberry	1 tablespoon	7
Vinegar, rice	1 tablespoon	2
Wasabi, powder	1/4 ounce	24
Worcestershire Sauce	1 teaspoon	5
Yeast, Bakers, active-dry	1/4 ounce	20
Yeast, Bakers, rapid rise	1/4 ounce	20

Crackers	Serving Size	Calories
Graham	2 full crackers	140
	1 cup crushed	55.3
Melba Toast, plain	1 round	11.7
Norwegian Flat Bread	1 each	21.2
Rye Krisp	2 triple crackers	45

Saltines	5 crackers	70
	1 oyster cracker	4.3
	1 cup crushed	303.8
Wasa rye crisp bread	1 each	36.6

Milk	Serving Size	Calories
Buttermilk, dry	1 tablespoon	25
Buttermilk, 1% fat	1 cup	99
Chocolate Milk, regular	1 cup	210
Chocolate Milk, low fat 2%	1 cup	180
Chocolate Milk, low fat 1%	1 cup	160
Chocolate Milk, fat free	1 cup	150
Coconut Milk, regular, canned	1 tablespoon	30
Coconut Milk, light, canned	1 tablespoon	10
Condensed Milk	1/3 cup	320
Cream, half & half	1 cup	315
Cream, 25% fat	1 cup	583
Cream, whipping, heavy	1 cup	821

Evaporated Milk, whole	1/2 cup	170
Evaporated Milk, skim	1/2 cup	100
Milk, whole	1 cup	157
Milk, 2% fat	1 cup	121
Milk, 1% fat	1 cup	102
Milk, fat-free or skim	1 cup	86
Sour Cream, regular	2 tablespoons (1 ounce)	61
Sour Cream, light	2 tablespoons (1 ounce)	40
Sour Cream, fat-free	2 tablespoons (1 ounce)	20
Soy Milk	1 cup	79
Yogurt, Plain (regular)	1 cup	139
Yogurt, Plain (low fat)	1 cup	144
Yogurt, Plain (non fat)	1 cup	127

Eggs	Serving Size	Calories
Egg, large	1	75
Egg White, large	1 egg white	17
Egg Whites	1 cup egg whites	121
Egg Yolk, large	1	59

| Egg Substitute, liquid | 1/4 cup (equals 1 egg) | 25 |

Butter/Oil	Serving Size	Calories
Butter, regular	1 teaspoon	33
	1 tablespoon	100
	1/4 cup	400
	1/2 cup - 1 stick or cube (4 oz)	813
Butter, whipped	1 tablespoon	67
Ghee	1 ounce	249
Lard	1 tablespoon	115
	1 cup	1849
Oils - canola, corn, olive, safflower, soybean, sesame, grapeseed	1 teaspoon	40
	1 tablespoon	120
Oils - almond, walnut, hazelnut, sesame, truffle (white & black)	1 tablespoon	120

Peanut Butter, smooth	2 tablespoons	188
Peanut Butter, chunk style	2 tablespoons	188
Peanut Butter, reduced fat	2 tablespoons	180
Shortening, vegetable, regular, or butter flavor	1 tablespoon	110

Flours	Serving Size	Calories
All-Purpose Flour, unsifted	1 cup (120 gm)	400
	1/4 cup (30 gm)	100
	1 tablespoon (7.5 gm)	25
Bread Flour	1 cup	495
Cake Flour	1 cup	400
Corn (Semolina) Flour	3 tablespoons	110
Oat Flour, blend	1 cup	390
Potato Starch	1 tablespoon	40
Rice Flour	1 cup	560
Rye Flour, light	1 cup	374
Rye flour, dark	1 cup	440

Soy Flour. low fat	1 cup	287
Tapioca Flour	1/4 cup	100
Whole Grain Flour	1 cup	407
Fruits	**Serving Size**	**Calories**
Apple, fresh	1 medium	81
Apple cider, canned or bottled	6 ounces	85
Apple juice, unsweetened	6 ounces	87
Applesauce, canned, unsweetened	1/2 cup	56
Apricots, fresh	3 medium	51
Avocado, fresh	1 ounce	46
	1/4 medium	55
	1 medium	324
	1/2 cup, pureed	185
Banana, fresh	1 medium	105
	1/2 cup mashed	104

Blackberries, fresh	1/2 cup	37
Blueberries, fresh	1/2 cup	41
Boysenberries, fresh	1/2 cup	37
Cantaloupe, fresh	1/2 medium	94
	1/2 cup cubed	29
Cherries, sweet w/o pits, fresh	1/2 cup	52
Cherries, sour w/o pits, fresh	1/1 cup	39
Cherries, dried, tart	1/4 cup	140
Cherry, Maraschino	1 each	8
Cranberries, whole, fresh	1/2 cup	23
Cranberry Juice, cocktail	6 ounces	110
Cranberry Sauce, canned, sweetened	1/2 cup	209
Currents, dried	1 cup	408

Dates, pitted, fresg	1 cup pitted & chopped	502
	1 date	23
Figs, fresh	1 small	30
	1 medium	37
	1 large	47
Figs, dried	10 figs	477
Grapefruit, pink or red	1/2 medium	60
	1/2 cup sections w/juice	43
Grapefruit Juice, fresh	6 ounces	72
Grapes, fresh	1 cup	62
Grape Juice, canned or bottled	1 cup	154
Honeydew Melon, fresh	1/10 medium	46
	1/2 cup cubed	30
Kiwifruit, fresh	1 medium	46
	1 large	55
Lemon, fresh	1 medium	17
	1 large	25

Lemon Peel (Zest)	1 teaspoon	0
	1 tablespoon	0
Lemon Juice, fresh	1 tablespoon	4
	1/2 cup	30
Lime	1 medium	20
Lime Juice, fresh	1 tablespoon	4
	1/2 cup	33
Mango, fresh	1 medium	135
	1/2 cup sliced	54
Nectarines, fresh	1 medium	67
	1/2 cup sliced	34
Orange Juice, fresh	6 ounces	83
Orange Juice, Fresh	1/4 cup	27.6
Orange Juice, canned or bottled	6 ounces	78
Peach, fresh	1 medium	37
Peach, canned in light syrup	halves	68
Peach, canned in water	halves	29

Pear, fresh	1 medium or large	98
Pear, canned in light syrup	halves	72
Pear Nectar	halves	62
Pineapple, fresh, trimmed	1 slice (3/4" thick)	42
	1/2 cup diced	39
Pineapple canned water-packed	1 cup (crushed, sliced or chunks)	78.7
	1 slice or ring	15
Pineapple Juice, canned or bottled	6 ounces	104
Plum, fresh, pitted	1 ounce	16
Pomegranate, fresh	1 pomegranate (3-3/8" dia)	105
Pomegranate Juice	8 ounces	150
Prickly Pear, fresh	1 medium	42
Prunes, dried	10 each	201

Prune Juice, canned	6 ounces	136
Raisins, seedless	1/2 cup (not packed)	219
	1/2 cup (packed)	249
Raspberries, fresh	1/2 cup	31
Raspberry Juice, canned or bottled	8 ounces	120
Strawberries, fresh	8 berries	50
	1/2 cup	23
Tangerine, fresh	1 medium	37
Watermelon, fresh	1/2 cup diced	25

Herbs & Spices	Serving Size	Calories
Allspice, ground	1 teaspoon	5
	1 tablespoon	16
Basil, Fresh	2 tablespoons	1
Basil, Dried	1 teaspoon	2
Bay Leaf	1 teaspoon	2
	1 tablespoon	6

Capers, drained	1 tablespoon	2
Chili Powder	1 teaspoon	6
	1 tablespoon	24
Cinnamon, ground	1 teaspoon	6
	1 tablespoon	18
Cloves, ground	1 teaspoon	7
	1 tablespoon	21
Coriander Leaf, dried	1 teaspoon	2
Coriander Seed	1 tablespoon	5
	1 tablespoon	15
Cumin Seeds	1 tablespoon	23
Curry Powder	1 teaspoon	6
	1 tablespoon	20
Dill Weed, dried	1 teaspoon	3
	1 tablespoon	8
Dill Weed, fresh	1 cup sprigs	4
Dill Seeds	1 tablespoon	20
Garlic Powder	1 teaspoon	9
	1 tablespoon	28

Garlic Salt	1 teaspoon	3
Ginger, ground	1 teaspoon	6
	1 tablespoon	19
Ginger Root	1 ounce	20
	5 slices	8
Marjoram, dried	1 teaspoon	2
	1 tablespoon	5
Nutmeg, ground	1 teaspoon	11
	1 tablespoon	37
Oregano, dried	1 teaspoon	6
	1 tablespoon	18
Paprika	1 teaspoon	6
	1 tablespoon	20
Parsley, fresh	10 sprigs	4
	1/2 cup, chopped	10
Parsley, dried	1 tablespoons	4
Pepper, Black, ground	1 tablespoon	16
Pepper, Red Or Cayenne, ground	1 tablespoon	17
	1 tablespoon	21

Pepper, White

Rosemary, fresh	1 tablespoon	2
Rosemary, dried	1 tablespoon	11
Saffron	1 teaspoon	2
Sage, ground	1 teaspoon	2
	1 tablespoon	6
Salt, iodized or non-iodized	1 teaspoon	0
	1 tablespoon	0
Thyme, dried	1 teaspoon	4
	1 tablespoon	12
Thyme, fresh	1 teaspoon	1

Lamb	Serving Size	Calories
Lamb, blade chop	1 chop	128
Lamb, ground	4 ounces	318.7
Lamb, loin chop (lean)	3 ounces	124

	Serving Size	Calories
Lamb, rib chop (lean)	3 ounces	136
Lamb, shoulder (lean)	3 ounces	116
Meats	**Serving Size**	**Calories**
Braunschweiger (liver sausage)	1 ounce	100
Deer, Tenderloin	3 ounces	127
Elk, Tenderloin	3 ounces	138
Pepperoni	1 ounces	130
Polish Kielbasa (Healthy Choice)	2 ounces	80
Smoked Sausage (Healthy Choice)	2 ounces	80
Smoked Kielbasa (Polish, Turkey & Beef)	2 ounces	127
Nuts/Seeds	**Serving Size**	**Calories**

Almonds, whole, dry roasted	1 each	6
	1 ounce	161
	1 cup, ground	546
	1 cup, whole	822
Almonds, sliced	1 cup	529
Almonds, slivered	1 cup	621
Brazilnuts, whole, shelled	1 ounce (6-8 nuts)	183
Brazilnuts, whole, shelled	1 cup	918
Caraway Seeds	1 teaspoon	7
	1 tablespoon	22.3
Cashews, dry roasted	1 ounce	162
	1 cup (halves & whole)	796
Filberts (hazelnuts), whole	1 each	8.7
	1 ounce	179
	1 cup	853
Filberts (hazelnuts), chopped	1 cup	727
Macadamia, whole & halves	1 ounce (10-12 nuts)	199

Peanuts, cooked & shelled	1 ounce	90.2
	1/2 cup	414
Peanuts, dry roasted	1 ounce	160
Peanut Butter, creamy or smooth	2 tablespoons	189
Peanut Butter, reduced-fat	2 tablespoons	100
Pecan, halves	1 ounce (20 nuts)	190
Pine Nuts	1 ounce	146
	1 tablespoon	51
Pistachios	1-ounce (47 nuts)	164
	1 cup	739
Poppy Seeds	1 teaspoon	14.9
	1 tablespoon	46.9
Sesame Seeds, toasted	1 teaspoon	10
	1 tablespoon	52

Sunflower Seeds, roasted, hulled and salted	1 ounce	87
Sunflower Seeds, oil roasted with salt	1 ounce	166
Walnuts	1-ounce (14 halves)	142
	1 cup (50 halves)	784.8
	1 cup (chopped or pieces)	770

Grains/Pasta	Serving Size	Calories
Barley, raw	1 ounce	100
	1 cup	651
Bulgur (Tabbouleh)	1 cup dry	479
	1 cup cooked	152
Couscous	1 cup dry	692
	1 cup cooked	201
Noodles (Chinese chow mein)	1 cup	237

Noodles (Japanese soba, somen, rice)	2 ounces dry	200
Pasta (egg noodles, linguine, macaroni, spaghetti, spials, lasagne, etc.)	2 ounces dry	212
Rice, arborio	3 tablespoons dry	150
	1 cup cooked	241
Rice, brown long-grain	1 cup dry	684
	1 cup cooked	216
Rice, white long grain (parboiled or instant)	1 cup dry	360
	1 cup cooked	161
Rice (glutinous or Sushi)	1 cup dry	685
	1 cup cooked	234
Rice, wild	1 cup raw	571
	1 cup cooked	166

Meats	Serving Size	Calories
Bacon, cured, raw	1 ounce	158

	1 thick slice (1.3 ounce)	174
Bacon, cooked	1 thin slice (.2 ounce)	27
	1 thick slice (.4 ounce)	58
Bacon Bits	1 tablespoon	30
Bacon Bits, Imitation	1 teaspoon	26
Bacon, Canadian style	1-ounce slice (unheated)	45
Bologna, pork	1 slice (1 ounce)	80
Bratwurst (fully cooked)	2-ounce link	170
Ham, cured (butt, lean)	3.5 ounces	159
Ham, fresh (lean)	1 ounce slice	45
Luncheon meat, beef/pork	1 ounce slice	76
Pork Chop, cooked and trimmed of fat		
center cut	2.5 ounces	166
top loin chops	3 ounces	171
rib chops	3 ounces	186

Pork Sausage	1 link (raw)	44
	1 patty (raw)	92
Pork Roast, cooked and boneless	3 ounces	165
Loin (tenderlooin) Roast	3 ounces	182
Rib Roast		
Spare Ribs, roasted	6 medium	396
Tenderloin Roast (lean and roasted)	3 ounces	130
	1 pound	740.8

White Meats	Serving Size	Calories
Chicken Broth or Stock, fat-free	1 cup	5
Chicken Breast (w/o skin)	1/2 breast	142
Chicken Leg (w/o skin)	1 leg or drumstick	76
Chicken Meat, roasted	1 cup (chopped or diced)	241
Chicken, whole, meat only, raw	2 pounds	1006

	Serving Size	Calories
Chicken Thigh (w/o skin)	1 thigh	109
Chicken Hotdog	1	116
Turkey breast, processed	1 ounce	51
Turkey breast, BBQ	3.5 ounce	135
Turkey breast, roasted	3.5 ounce	115
Turkey breast, smoked	3.5 ounce	120
Turkey breast, white meat, no skin	3 ounce	120
Turkey, dark meat, no skin	3 ounce	140
Turkey hot dog	1	102
Turkey, ground	4 ounces	169.9
	1 pound	675.9
Turkey Kielbasa, 95% fat free	2 ounces	70

Seafood	Serving Size	Calories
Anchovy Fillets	5 medium each (appx .7 oz)	42
Caviar	1 ounce	72

Clams, raw	1 each small	6.7
	1 each medium	10.7
	1 cup w/liquid	168
	9 large or 20 small	133
	1 pound w/shells	50.3
Clams, canned	1 cup w/liquid	236.8
Clams Juice, canned or bottled	1 tablespoon	0
	1 cup	4.8
Cod	3.5 ounces	85
Crab Meat, cooked (Dungeness, Blue, King & Lump)	3 ounces	90
	1 pound	391
	1 whole crab	139.7
Flounder/Sole	3.5 ounces	68
Grouper	3.5 ounces	87
Halibut	3 ounces	93.5
	6 ounces	187
	1/2 fillet	224
Lobster	1 ounce	33
	3.5 ounces	91

Mussels, w/o shells	1 ounce	24.4
	3 ounces	73
Oysters, Pacific raw	1 medium	40.5
	4 ounces	81
Oysters, Eastern raw	1 medium	8.2
Red Snapper	3.5 ounces	93
Salmon, Atlantic	3 ounces	155.6
Salmon, Atlantic	1 pound	612.5
	2 pounds	1225
Salmon, smoked	3.5 ounces	176
Salmon, pink canned	3 ounces	118
	1 can (14 3/4-oz)	630.5
Scallops, raw	2 large or 5 small	26.4
	3 ounces	74.8
	1/2 pound	199.4
Shrimp or Prawns	1 small each	5.3
	1 medium each	6.4
	1 large	7.4
	3 ounces	90

Shrimp, canned & drained	1 ounce	25
Trout, Rainbow	3.5 ounces	195
Tuna, fresh	3.5 ounces	177
Tuna, solid white, canned in water	2 ounces 3-ounce can or pouch 7-ounce can or pouch	70 90 180

Snacks	Serving Size	Calories
Beef Jerky	1 piece	82
Popcorn, 94% fat free (average most brands)	1/2 (1.5 oz) microwave package 1 (3 oz) microwave package	130 260
Popcorn, popped without oil or butter	1 ounce dry or 1 quart popped	109

Sugars/Syrups	Serving Size	Calories
Corn Syrup, light	2 tablespoons	120
Honey	1 tablespoon	60

Molasses, dark, unsulphured	1 tablespoon	60
Sugar, granulated	1 teaspoon (level)	15
	1 tablespoon	46
	1 cup	770
	1 cube	9
	1 packet (2 ounces)	23
Sugar, Bakers or superfine	1 teaspoon	15
Sugar, brown	1 teaspoon	17
	1 tablespoon	41
	1/4 cup, packed	164
	1/2 cup, packed	328
Sugar, powdered or confectioners, unsifted	1 tablespoon	31
	1 cup	462
Syrup, Maple	1 tablespoon	50

Misc	Serving Size	Calories
Avocado Roll	1 roll (appx 6 to 7 pieces)	140

California Roll	1 roll (appx 6 to 7 pieces)	255
Cucumber Roll	1 roll (appx 6 to 7 pieces)	136
Philadelphia Roll (salmon, cream cheese, avocado)	1 roll (appx 6 to 7 pieces)	319
Salmon & Avocado	1 roll (appx 6 to 7 pieces)	304
Shrimp Tempura roll	1 roll (appx 6 to 7 pieces)	508
Spicy Tuna Roll	1 roll (appx 6 to 7 pieces)	290
Spider Roll (fried soft-shell crab):	1 roll (appx 6 to 7 pieces)	317
Abalone Tuna	1 piece over rice	45

Bluefin Tuna	1 piece over rice	50
Flounder	1 piece over rice	43
Octopus	1 piece over rice	53
Salmon	1 piece over rice	56
Salmon Roe	1 piece over rice	39
Sea Bass	1 piece over rice	41
Sea Urchin	1 piece over rice	64
Squid	1 piece over rice	43
Tamago (Japanese Omelet)	1 piece over rice	75
Yellowtail Tuna	1 piece over rice	51
Edamame (Green beans)	1/2 cup	100
Pickled Ginger	1 serving (.5 ounce)	9
Toasted Nori Seaweed	1 sheet	10

Miso Soup (no tofu added)	1 cup	40
Seasoned Sushi Rice (cooked with rice vinegar and sugar)	1 cup	170

Veggies	Serving Size	Calories
Arugula, raw	1 pound	104
	1 oz	7
	1/2 cup	2
Artichoke, globe	1 medium (11.3 oz)	60
	1 large (14.3 oz)	76
Artichoke hearts, canned & marinated	3.5 oz	225
Asparagus, raw	1 pound	54
	4 spears	13
Beans, green (fresh)	1/2 cup	22
Beans, green (canned) & drained	1/2 cup	23
Beans, black, canned	1/2 cup	100
	15-ounce can	200

Beans, Garbanzo (chick peas), canned	1/2 cup	80
	15.5-ounce can	160
Beans, Kidney, canned	1/2 cup	104
Beans, White, canned	1/2 cup	110
	15-ounce can	220
Beans, lentils, cooked/boiled	1/2 cup	115
Beans, Lima, cooked/boiled	1/2 cup	104
Beans, refried, canned, regular	1/2 cup	121
Beans, refried vegetarian	1/2 cup	70
Beans, navy, cooked	1/2 cup	129
Beets	2 medium	71
	1/2 cup sliced	30
Broccoli	1 medium stalk or spear	42
	1/2 cup chopped	12
Brussel Sprouts	1 sprout	8

Cabbage, Chinese raw	1/2 cup shredded	5
Cabbage, green raw	1/2 cup shredded	28
Cabbage, red raw	1/2 cup shredded	10
Carrot, raw	1 baby	5
	1 medium	25
	1 large	30
Cauliflower	1 medium head	144
	1 floweret	3
Celery	1 large stalk or rib	9
	1 medium stalk or rib	6
	1 small stalk or rib	2
Chiles, green, canned	2 tablespoons	10
Corn, fresh, yellow or white, raw	1/2 cup kernels	66
	1 medium ear (90 g)	80
	1 large ear (146 g)	155
Corn, cream style	1/2 cup	93
Cucumber	1 medium to large	39

Eggplant, raw	1 medium	27
Endive	1/2 cup chopped	4
	1 head	86
Garlic	1 clove	4
Greens (Collards), raw	1/2 cup chopped	6
Greens (Collards), boiled drained	1/2 cup chopped	17
Jicama (Yam Bean Tuber)	1 ounce	12
	1 pound untrimmed	170
Lettuce, Bibb, Boston or Butterhead	1 head 7.75 oz)	21
Lettuce, Iceberg	1 medium head (1.25 lbs)	70
Lettuce, Coss or Romaine	1 inner leaf (.4 oz)	2
Mushrooms, (white or brown) raw	5 medium	20
	1/2 cup pieces or slices	15
Mushrooms (Portabella) raw	1 large cap	20
Mushroom Pieces, canned & drained	1/2 cup	21

Okra, raw	8 pods	36
Okra, cooked/boiled & drained	8 pods	27
Okra, frozen	10-oz package	85
Onion, yellow, white, red, & sweet	1 large	65
	1 medium	40
	1/2 cup, chopped	30
	1 tablespoons, chopped	4
	1 thin slice	4
	1 medium slice (1/8")	6
	1 large slice (1/4")	16
Onions, green	1 cup chopped	32
	1 large	8
	1 medium (4 1/8" long)	5
	1 small (3" long)	2
Onion, dried or dehydrated	1 tablespoon	16
	1/4 cup	45
Peas, green, snap	1/2 cup	67
	1 cup	110
Peas, black-eyed (cooked)	1/2 cup	99
Peas, split peas	1/4 cup dry	110

Peas, Snow or Sugar	1/2 cup	34
Pepper, bell	1 medium	35
	2 tablespoons minced	1
	1/2 cup chopped	12
Pepper, red roasted	7 ounce jar	50
Pepper, chile	1 pepper	20
Pepper, chipotle in adobe sauce, canned	2 tablespoons	15
Potato. baked with skin	1 small (4.9 oz)	128
	1 medium (6.1 oz)	161
	1 large (10.5 oz)	278
Potato, Baby Red-Skinned, boiled	4 ounces	86
Potato, sweet, baked with skin	1 medium (6.3 oz)	136
Pumpkin, canned	1/2 cup	40

Radish	1 medium (.2 oz)	1
	1 large (.3 oz)	1
	1/2 cup slices (2 oz)	9 to 10
Rutabaga	1 cup, cubed	25
Sauerkraut, canned, solids & liquid	1/2 cup drained	27
Shallots, raw	1 tablespoon	7.2
Spinach, raw	1 leaf (.4 oz)	2
	1 bunch (12 oz)	78
Squash, Acorn, raw	1 medium (15.2 oz)	172
	1 cup cubes (4.9 oz)	56
Squash, Butternut, raw	1 cup cubes (4.9 oz)	63
Squash, Zucchini, raw	1 small (4.2 oz)	19
	1 medium (6.9 oz)	31
	1 large (11.4 oz)	52
Tomato, whole, raw	1 medium	26
Tomato, whole, raw	1 large	38
Tomato, Cherry, raw	1 cherry	4
Tomato, Cherry, raw	5 each	10

Tomato, Italian or Plum	1 each	13
Tomatoes, whole canned	1/2 cup	24
	1 cup	48
	14.5 oz can	15
	28 oz can	35
Tomatoes, diced or crushed	14.5-ounce can - 3 (1/2 cup) servings	87.5
	28-ounce can - 7 (1/2 cup) servings	175
Tomato Paste, canned	2 tablespoons	30
	6-ounce can	150
Tomato Sauce, canned	2 tablespoons	30
	1 cup	73.5
	6-ounce can	150
Tomato juice	1 cup (8 ounces)	41
Tomatillo	1 medium	10.88
Vegetable Cocktail Juice (V8 Juice)	1 cup	46
	5.5-ounce can	30

| Water chestnuts | 4 water chesthuts | 35 |
| | 5-ounce can | 75 |

Note from the author:

I wish all of you the best of luck. I know
that you will have just as much success
with this as I did. I look forward to
hearing all of your success stories.
Please feel free to email me
mariaphelps5@yahoo.com